40 Steps to Make Any Woman Have an Orgasm.

How to Start the Orgasmic Process. The Ultimate Guide to Female Orgasm.

DAVID GOMADZA

www.twofuture.world

DEDICATION

To all women out there.

TABLE OF CONTENTS

INTRODUCTION 1

AROUSAL AS THE ULTIMATE PIECE OF THE PUZZLE OF CREATION. 3

ATTENTION AS THE KEY TO ORGASM AND CREATION 6

ORGASM AS A PREDEFINED PARAMETER 13

HOW THE VAGINA PREPARES FOR ORGASM 16

THE ULTIMATE RECIPE TO GET A WOMAN AN ORGASM OF THE CENTURY 18

THE RHYTHMIC SYSTEM OF THE VAGINA 21

NEEDED PARAMETERS FOR VAGINAL ORGASM 22

THE VAGINA'S COLOR CODE FOR STAGES OF AROUSAL. 24

WHAT IS A VAGINA AND WHAT IS IT THAT IT DOES? 26

THE IMPORTANCE OF THE VAGINAL HOLD AND WHAT CAN BE DONE TO AFFECT THIS CONDITION. 28

WHAT CAN BE DONE TO IMPROVE ON THE LAST KNOWN BEST ORGASMIC CLIMAX POINT? 29

WHAT PARTS DOES A VAGINA HAVE AND THEIR ROLE IN ORGASM? 32

HOW THE VAGINA ACTUALLY PERFORMS AN ORGASM. 34

PROCESSES INSIDE THE VAGINA CALLED SQUANKS. 40

SPECIFIC QUESTIONS POSED TO THE VAGINA REGARDING ORGASM. 42

GIVING WOMEN A SECOND CHANCE BY CREATING A BEST KNOW GOOD GONFIGURATION 44

A QUICK LOOK AT MALE EJACUALTION 45

ORGASM AND EJACULATION AS THE ANSWER TO CREATION AND GOD'S PLAN 46

WOMEN GET A DESIGNER VAGINA USING THESE CODES 48

40 Steps to Make Any Woman Have an Orgasm.

MEN GET A DESIGNER PENIS USING THESE CODES. 49

40 Steps to Make Any Woman Have an Orgasm.

ACKNOWLEDGMENTS

Tomorrow's World Order.
A better world for all.

INTRODUCTION

How the brain prepares and process sex
start.arousal.sex.penetration.climax.ejaculation.end

send correct signals to all body parts involved
1] send arousal stimuli to the appropriate regions of the body of a man.

2] send arousal stimuli to correct corresponding nerves.

3] send arousal stimuli to correct end points.

4] send arousal stimuli to correct nerve ends and corresponding nerve receptors where nerve receptors = nerve impulse at correct point - nerve stimuli that triggers it.

5] send correct anatomical entities to their corresponding places and start the actual arousal.

6] send nerve impulses to nerve receptors [where nerve receptors are the same as the desired targets] i.e. if you send correct nerve stimuli but to wrong nerve receptors then you won't get the desired outcome that means you must always send the correct nerve stimuli to the correct nerve receptors.

7] once all done now start the stimuli envisage process where the nerve stimuli is unpackaged and sorted into correct nerve stimuli receptors.

Once that is done now trigger the nerve response stimuli agents [these unmask the nerve stimuli identifying each and every one of the nerve stimuli; their function and the desired outcome intended.

Now ask what if this is the intended outcome them what?

Now initiate the nerve stimuli reaction response where each of the nerve stimuli is matched to its nerve response and the results noted.

Now trigger the reaction mechanism in which each nerve stimuli action is compared to the outcome and if correct then schedule for release [NB each nerve stimuli are and acts in line to the rest of the body system for a coordinated and effective response.]

What if we introduce something that does not give us the desired outcome then what?

If we are to say that if X is the same as Y why then should we not expect Y if we introduce X.

If we are to expect Y after introducing X then Y depend on X but what if Y is not achieved by the introduction of X. Can X need something else for us to get the desired outcome of Y.

I   f so then what is X + x = Y

This is our working assumption that if X + X = Y then we can easily get the outcome we want if we know what is X and what is x.

If we are to tell everyone what we want to do then everyone must know what that means and how they expect that to be so.

AROUSAL AS THE ULTIMATE PIECE OF THE PUZZLE OF CREATION.

Now ask what is the right stimuli to enact an arousal effect on sight of
a beautiful woman?
Arousal is the ultimate piece to the puzzle of creation.
Arousal is the end goal in itself in that it must lead to mating or else
there is no humanity.
Arousal is the hinge pin to the puzzle of creation. If there was no
arousal then there wouldn't be expected to be humanity.
This is true in that arousal is the trigger of creation, without arousal
men would not find women attractive and therefore would not need
the male [make love according to the human dictionary]
If we are to ask what women want its simply the attraction and
attention they get from men [nowadays from other women]
It is this attention that motivates women to be what they want.
It's this attention that makes women be women.
It's this attention that makes women ovulate.
If there was no attention then there wouldn't be ovulation [women
only ovulate when the attention they get reach a certain satisfactory
level.
If the level is not reached that woman will not ovulate.
These are the simple facts of life nonetheless less paid attention to.
Now let's delve deeper into the female biological clock.
If we are to ask the female biological clock what makes a woman horny
it will simply reply with a one-word answer; attention paid to it.
This is all what it takes.

Now ask yourself what can a woman do to increase the chances of getting so much attention that she literally ovulates on the spot?
A woman can easily seduce a man so that all that a man wants is to give her attention.
[attraction is a mutual feeling. That means that the woman must be attractive or possess something that man wants likewise the man must be attractive two for it to work both ways.
Now what happens to ovulation if the woman does not get enough attention to trigger ovulation.
A woman needs at least 90% of daily attention dosage to start ovulating.
Women must feel loved, wanted and needed to start ovulating or have signs that mimic ovulation.
If we are to ask the female body what makes it ovulate it will simply say it's because of the attention it gets during the day and how it is stored in the body.
If attention is wasted and not kept properly then when it comes to summoning the ingredients simply because they have been stored in the wrong places or lost altogether.
Now let's look into how women store attention throughout the day.
Women save all feelings of being loved, wanted and needed on their private parts mainly inside the vagina.
But there are specific locations in the vagina for these attention feelings.
Inside the vagina a closer look.
Now let's examine the vagina.
Let's look inside to see exactly what happens to everything that occurs throughout the day.
We can easily identify the places where the attention feelings are stored by asking why we need them in the first place. Woman need attention stimuli in order for their bodies to release eggs that is ovulate.
If a woman feels loved cared for and needed she will release an egg so that the man feels loved in return this is how nature is.
It is a thank you for giving me attention in return have an egg. That said now let's delve deeper into ovulation cycle.
Women ovulate to release their selves when loved as eggs. You love me that much then I will give you my egg in return to care and love even more.
Now let's ask the universe what it feels about the laws of attraction.
The universe understands the laws of attention when two planets,

things, humans etc. attract to each other than reciprocity is the results.
Reciprocity means that two entities have come into an agreement that
they both find each other every attractive regardless of what others
think about this mutual agreement.
Now let's pose the universe somewhat if questions.
If we ask the universe what it thinks about mutual attraction this is its
reply.
Mutual attraction is a common attraction goal that makes two entities
agree to something that they find of common interest.
If we are to ask what this means then the universe might reply
What two identifies as attraction means they feel attracted to that and
as such must first agree to it and give testimony to it.
It is this testimony that makes it possible to mutual agree in the first
place.

ATTENTION AS THE KEY TO ORGASM AND CREATION

Now let's pose the universe another interesting question.

If we are to ask the universe what is attention then this is the reply:

attention is attraction from sight, smell, taste, vision imaginary included

attention is love at first sight attention is deception [where your eyes deceives you]

attention is arrogance [where you think you can get anything]

attention is envy

attention is greedy [wanting everything at any cost]

attention is seduction [thinking you can do anything that moves]

attention is lust

 attention is gloat [loving someone's else]

attention is religious [you worship the someone for that time]

attention is devotion

attention is lust plus sin put together

attention is jealous

attention is speed dating without the sex

attention is enormous range [if you lust for someone seeing them with another trigger

range in you

attention is kind

attention is cheap in that it does cost nothing to ogle a woman

attention is attention [attention means giving someone attention]

attention rocks

attention steal
attention rides
attention stirs up
attention dashes failure [no room for failing when attention is in play
attention overpowers
attention overrides [cancels objection commands all at once]
attention reverberates meaning energy is not lost but bounces off from one entity to the other
attention delivers and never fails [when you give a woman attention other thing being equal then the answer is yes.]
attention is king
attention is holy
attention is divine
attention is pride
attention is master
attention is lord
attention is everything all you need to do is give attention to something and that something obeys you
attention is duress
attention is ogliberant meaning it can always be relied upon to deliver results
attention is solemn
attention is endurance in itself
attention is completeness
attention is joy
attention is a gift
attention is wealth
attention is rock solid state
attention gets results
attention breeds yes
attention rewards with yes
attention influences decisions
attention targets results
attention is results
attention is holy even the angels bow to attention
attention propels progress
attention gives power
attention retains power
attention reattracts
attention restores

attention matures
attention merits greatness
attention revolves around success
attention is success
attention is key to progress
attention is master of ceremony
attention dictates pace
attention dictates progress
attention is holy even the gods pay attention to each other
attention is the final product
attention is the final closure
attention is the only sales pitch worth it
attention closes deals
attention gets things done
attention encompasses everyone
 attention depowers those who don't understand
it
attention renders evil useless in case of its absence
attention builds lives
attention builds humanity [if men did not give woman attention that
would have meant no mating and no births
attention means liking something enough to make it matter to you
anything you give attention to means it's important to you therefore
matters to you
attention is the word for wealth seekers
attention is the word for love seekers
anything you give attention to must obey according to the laws of the
universe
attention breeds love
attention breeds results
attention rewards persistence
attention is persistence
attention and attention = greatness
anything you pay attention to will give you its best
women if you give them attention they will give you their best in eggs
The universe if you pay it attention will give you its best its miniature
version.
attention is the language of the gods
attention is the love of the universe
attention is the love of creation

attention is the love of love
attention breeds love
attention breeds honesty
attention is pledging one's self
attention is loyalty to anything you pay attention to
attention means completeness
attention means devotion
attention is truthful
attention means honesty
attention means full cooperation
attention means surrender to
attention means evolution
attention means solidarity with
attention means pure
attention means pure and holy
attention means welcome
attention means endure
attention means persevere
attention means amplitude
attention means respect
attention means dishonesty if omitted
attention means revered
attention means honest if acted upon
attention means attention plus the added commitment
attention means grasping the idea and what is needed
attention means challenging everything
attention means working hypothesis
attention means everything right
attention means setting your goal high
attention means feeling loved
attention means hoping to get results in that paying attention means
doing what is needed to achieve the goal
attention means getting everything right first time
attention means acting promptly in that if you pay attention then
chances are that you know what can go wrong and how to fix it
attention means getting things sorted fast
attention means responding fast
attention means asking the right questions
attention means doing the right things
attention means deserving the best

attention means asking for the right price of something
attention means doing everything according to what is needed
attention means connecting everything properly
attention means doing everything right
attention means being on schedule
attention means repairing everything on time
attention means focusing
attention means inspecting correctly
attention means writing correctly
attention means understanding correctly first time
attention means no room for errors
attention means going by the book [book are rules and regulations]
attention means showing you know and your interest
attention means resolving issues fast
attention means admitting to your weakness
attention means the need to be supported
attention means the need to safeguard your interests
 attention means doing everything right as scheduled
attention means resolving issues amicably
attention means aware of surroundings
attention means resolving issues and fixing future ones
attention means anticipation meaning planning ahead
attention means focusing on something
attention means challenging status quo
attention means getting addressed on issues that matter
attention means absorbing the truth
attention means relating to the issue as you will have a clear idea of
the problem
attention means seeking nothing but the truth
attention means getting noticed for your contributions
attention means resolving issues that can impact future operations
attention means attention with the great extra care
attention means omitting waste
attention means resolving all issues
attention means acknowledging the truth
attention means resolving all your issues
attention means acknowledging the truth
attention means resolving all your issues
attention means analyzing everything
attention means getting facts right

attention means seeking the truth in terms of operations
attention results in positive change
attention results in time saving
attention results in good time keeping
attention results in good time management
attention results in cost saving
attention results in optimal use of something
attention means acting prompt
attention means reserved
attention means chosen
attention means picked out of all
attention means resulting in progress
attention means reserved opinion
attention means aware and induced to act
attention means joined in that you will form partnership at the end if there is mutual agreement
attention means seeking success
attention means getting things done
attention means authorizing someone and something
attention means getting someone trust if you are on the receiving end
attention means getting honored
attention means getting trusted
attention means getting revered
attention means mutual cooperation
attention means amused
attention means getting noticed
attention means targeted work
attention means using the correct techniques
attention means choosing the right path
attention means correcting your mistakes
attention means covering your tracks [to avoid mistakes and in advance - proactive]
attention means highlighting the truth
attention means fixing the right problems
attention means sorting out any mess
attention means replacing all the defected
attention means asking the truth
attention means challenging the norm
attention means doing the right thing
attention is attention with the added commitment and perseverance

attention is attention without the ass licking
attention means no bribery
attention means no corruption for what you see is what you get
attention deserves to be given attention to attention is for the clever and outright perfect
attention sets you apart from the rest
attention means attention with the time management and keeping
attention is all what is needed to conquer in life
the most successful billionaires, millionaires, politicians etc. all pay attention to attention

ORGASM AS A PREDEFINED PARAMETER

As going back to the theme of the brain reading chapter we can conclude that arousal between a man and a woman is not that complicated because it follows a predefined pattern that to master arousal all things being equal you simply need to know the following facts

1] woman like attention but not from everyone you must possess

i] charm

ii] charisma

iii] trust

iv] honesty

v] handsomeness

vi] money to some extent

to woo a woman to bed but this is the outward appearance.

What if we are to ask what goes inside the body is the answer the same as above?

Now let look again what happens inside a woman's vagina during arousal.

when the vagina is aroused it sends chemical signals to the correct sockets inside it

Chemical 1

This triggers production of the first-class hormones. First class hormones ask questions where pointing to place and time inside the vagina.

Chemical 2

These trigger production of second-class hormones. Second class hormones ask two questions;

a] how to do it if its inside vagina

b] when the time

If we have to answer we can easily answer with a map pinned on a clock

Just put a pin on when on the clock and diagram of how we can do that.

Chemical 3

These trigger the production of third-class hormones. What is the effect of doing all this.

To answer we must go back to the pre-defined parameters and ask if we are to increase third class hormones then what will the body do in response?

Chemical 4

These trigger the production of fourth class which seeks to solve any problems within the already predefined parameters.

If we are to act on these we can simply ask why if its predefined then why it is not happening now?

If we are to deal with these we can easily say what is not going what it is supposed to do.

The answer will be straight forward.

Chemical 5

These trigger the production of firth class hormones that asks so many questions at the same time just before the release of sex hormones

1] what if we increase everything but one what happens

2] what if we miss one but everything what happens

3] what do we do when all is activated but none acting upon sex hormones

4] if we are to deactivate all what then

 5] if we are to ask what can we do

6] if we are to accentuate everything what then

7] if we are to go ahead what can be the outcome if one fails

8] can we do all this over and over again with the same results

9] can we honestly say that we can prepare the body before release of sex hormones

10] can we control the outcome and stop everything within time of release of sex hormones and with what effect

11] can we add something else to spice things up and what is it

12] can we honestly say that we can prepare the body just before sex hormones release

what if we are to reduce everything in quantities will we get the desired effect if we have everything in order can we still or should we still expect the same outcome

if we are to add something then what is it

if we are to remove something then what is it

if we honestly trigger huge arousal what is the best recipe in a woman?

if we ask the vagina what to expect during arousal what can it say?

The vagina will answer that hell on earth no one has the biggest task to prepare for an orgasm than me even the brain does less preparation to think than me. I of all the organs including the heart do a lot of preparation to such an extent that in most cases intercourse happen before I finished no wonder why some women cannot orgasm.

HOW THE VAGINA PREPARES FOR ORGASM

Here is a list of all the things i must do first before orgasm

1] breath sharply to activate rhythms

2] spark inside like car sparking plugs

3] emerge saliva all over myself for lubrication

4] tear small pieces through electromagnetic wave internisonents where electromagnetic waves stretch and tear the inside of the vagina muscle so that there are slight cuts that give women arousal [72839848682]

if these cuts are missing, not pronounced etc. then everything will have to be repeated. But how these are made in the first place.

They form as vagina is stretched in relation to electromagnetic wave internisonents as described above.

The vibrations cause tiny vagina ulceration.

These then stretch to make things even more pronounced during vagina rhythmic phase.

The greater the vaginal rhythms the greater the ulcerations and the orgasm act.

Now let's tiny and go stage by stage not because that is easy but we must try to understand why women orgasm in the first place.

Vagina is created to ulcerate, vibrate, squit, squim, squam 72983868482, squim 729836489828, squimsh 72839868480, squoimsh 72859868483, squants 72869848380, squonts 72898483826, squantws 72869848328, squartzs 72869848382, squintzs 72869848321, squintmts 72869848320, squantzrs 7286984880, squartzzs 72836898464, squartzms 72869848321 [difference is in rythms per second], squrtzzst

72869848321 [difference is in rhythms per seconds x vibrations per minute]

Above all these must be in sequence for example if there is not squintzs that means everything ese that relies on this will be missing

We can tell that these are a lot of tasks for a vagina but how do these get activated?

By the woman or the attention?

We can tell that most of these are activated by the attention given rather than by the woman herself.

Attention is responsible for 90% of the activates that happen in the vagina for a woman to orgasm but if we ask what kind of attention is needed for each of these to be activated in the vagina we can see that for most it's the same kind of attention but at varying rythms and frequencies and vibrations.

That said that means it's not very hard to make a woman orgasm because you first need to be consistent in giving her attention.

THE ULTIMATE RECIPE TO GET A WOMAN AN ORGASM OF THE CENTURY

Now let's look at the ultimate recipe to get a woman an orgasm of the century.

1] Look at her in the eyes first and enter the spirit world with her by constantly eyeing her especially the right eye with your left eye.

2] Touch the top of her right hand once with your left hand

3] Ask what if and stop

4] Ask if then then what and stop

5] Look at her in the eyes and whisper her name first and ask what if and stop

6] Ask if she respond to you but don't expect an answer.

7] Ask if she knew all this and stop

8] Ask if she has experience and stop

9] Ask if she find but don't finish the line instead try to kiss her on the cheek but again stop this time hold her left hand and kiss it passionate and curse [damn woman why everything is like slow] and establish eye contact - your left eye in her right eye - smile very much and release all air inside you

10] kiss her forehead and say sorry you are fast I thought you are slow [but with enthusiasm] say you are the fastest but stop

11] Check your hand wrist watch and look away

12] Ask what time she think it is actually saying guess? Now keep quiet and just listen to her as if you are cooking a pressure cooker meal.

13] Check time one more time and frown but say something else nothing to do with you.

14] Now pat her back earnestly and start stroking her left hand all the way from the armpit to the finger tips and each time ask how fast this can be but ask as if you are asking how fast you can stroke her arm and nothing to do with sex.

15] Suggest you stroke faster as a question.

16] Say food is ready but don't salivate.

17]Say ok I am coming at the right time.

18] Pinch her inner left hand and say oh beautiful

19] Turn to check the inside palm of her hand and say oh beautiful I didn't know but stop

20] Say oh cheers I can celebrate to this

21] Imagine rubbing her nipples all at the same time and say simply put hot

22] Say if I didn't put then I would have understood why but stop

23] Now ask what's her favorite but stop

24] Look at her with cravings

25] Say how beautiful but and stop

26] Ask what if then stop

27] Ask what then and stop

28] Ask if then then what

29] Say very joyous if i had you i bet and stop

30] Now hold her left hand but quickly drop left hand and hold right hand

31] If you were ready this is how i would do things

32] If you were mine but stop

33] Not that you are not mine I am just saying that if I had power over you I would totally make everything fast and ready before you even say yes

34] If you knew how fast I am you would not even try to change but revamp everything to original way because this is how I changed mine in that case it's a mis-match

35] Unless then stop

36]I underestimated you. Did i?

37] I bet I did now I know pardon my French but I am ready and waiting is not my thing

38] I know we cannot wait that is what I am saying.

39] I am ready

40 Are you?

All this time override whatever she says with the next question. Don't answer long sentences, yes, no, can't happen unless if its mutual ok.

Try to memories all questions their job is to prepare the vagina fully ready for penetration.

Now initiate by a simple kiss on the cheek preferably right check.

Now always switch from right cheek to left cheek but after the questions never start on the left more from the right to the left only no matter what

THE RHYTHMIC SYSTEM OF THE VAGINA

Now let's look at the rhythmic system of the vagina.

The vagina if aroused goes in a rhythmic phase.

1]Pre-rhythmic

2]Rhythm

3] Post rhythm

4] Post and past rhythm

5] Repetition phase

6] Climax

7] Reset to original position preparing for next move

Now let's define every stage

1] Pre- rhythm

The vagina is in a quiet state. Everything is to its normal position.

But it takes only a fraction of a second for everything to start or even get to the next stage the rhythm stage.

Now this depends on woman and the attention given.

Now let's breakdown everything according to the above stages.

If we are to ask the vagina what it needs to kickstart everything then its response is simple.

It must get the right attention that triggers the right move rhythms.

A man or nowadays a woman must know how to give the vagina this attention.

There is no point in making love to a woman especially with orgasmic problems without knowing all these.

NEEDED PARAMETERS FOR VAGINAL ORGASM

A man or nowadays a woman must know how to give the vagina this attention.

There is no point in making love to a woman especially with orgasmic problems without knowing all these.

Therefore, we must define all the needed parameters one by one.

1] Arousal sticks these little sparks that are long hit the vagina inside to start the rhythmic stage.

Arousal sticks cracks the inside of the vagina inserting spark plugs so tiny no human eye can see these.

Once these are inserted into the inside of the vagina then the next stage is the need for the activation of the electromagnetic internisonent process where electromagnetic wave rhythmic movements causes the vagina to tear fast and start the arousal process.

Once that done we can then proceed to the next stage.

The next stage requires the spark plug inserted inside the vagina to be activated. The only way to this is to create a vacuum inside vagina. This allows the vagina to feel unwanted so that it contracts fast but attention from a man/woman [lesbian] send it expanding rapidly that it causes the inserted spark plugs to spark and as they spark this makes the vagina be activated electromagnetically as the sparks emits electromagnetic waves. This in turn means the start of electromagnetic internisonents where the vagina is ulcerated to such a point that arousal is inevitable and instant.

But not all this is repeated gives the same outcome.

All depends on the stage of arousal.
If we are to ask the vagina what stage of arousal are you at a given time the vagina must be able to tell us instantly. But how does the vagina know?

THE VAGINA'S COLOR CODE FOR STAGES OF AROUSAL.

How the vagina knows the stage of arousal.
1]The vagina characterises each stage by way of colours.
Green is the initial stage characterised by non-action but with the insertion of spark plugs. In this stage no action is evident all is saved for the next stage.
Yellow is the ready stage everything is ready but still no action.
Red this stage everything is ready but still no action. This is because attention has not reached 90% to effect change and a response.
Orange in this stage attention is about to hit 90% but it hasn't
Maroon attention is above 90% and everything has started but with mild rhythms.
Black everything is ready attention above 90% and everything has started the woman can feel the rhythms but cannot maintain the arousal.
Black diamond shinning black is when everything is so pronounced that a woman can easily orgasm but one thing is missing.
Black-red hottest stage everything is to highest levels attention is above 99.9999% the missing thing is love has just been added but hasn't activated enough to be felt.
Black-red-yellow the woman is about to orgasm fast and strong but one more ingredient is missing. The missing ingredient is a slap on the clit painful or not matters little. The clit has spark plugs that must be activated as well. A slap on her clit sparks the already ready spark plugs to send her to the moon and back.

Now if a man has given a woman enough attention asked the correct questions all 40 and took her through all the vagina colour codes then the woman must orgasm this is because these are pre-defined parameters and must work.
Now let's look at the hottest vagina colour code.
Black-red-yellow-black
This is the ultimate colour code for all woman's orgasm. Tell your woman this colour code just before orgasm.
Whisper in her ear
Black-red-yellow-black babe! repeat as needed.
Or just say 72869848382 repeatedly or give this code a name and call her just before orgasm.

WHAT IS A VAGINA AND WHAT IS IT THAT IT DOES?

Now if we are to ask the vagina what makes it what it is then the answer is that it makes woman experience the ultimate pleasure there is more than most men if it is at the right time.

But we must ask a lot of questions before we can say for sure that we know the vagina or know to make a woman orgasm any time.

First, we must ask what is a vagina once that is answered we must also ascertain what it is that the vagina does.

If we are to ask the vagina about the vagina. The vagina must answer us honestly for us to know.

A vagina is the most secretive organ that is hard to see for most men. Most even married rarely see what the vagina looks like because women tend to hide this as a way of seducing men. Men would love to kiss, caress, play with the vagina and fuck it hard if possible but women want to use it to attract men. Even when married women tend to starve men of the sight of the vagina.

Men love to look at the vagina as this gives them instant erection but how is this so?

The vagina shape is of a trapezoidal that means a purse or a pocket that if seen by a man will lock into the hard stimuli sockets of the man's brain to send hard erection signals to the penis resulting in an instant arousal and penial erection.

Once again this is not by chance but through pre-defined coordinates.

A man gets arousal just from the sight of a vagina just as a woman also measure the man's shaft and if it fits inside their man's shaft sockets in the brain they will receive instant arousal with a mild ejection of vaginal fluids.

If we are to show woman and erect penis and a man a vagina showing all corners they both are said to have an orgasm. This is because when the two happen at the same time they are both to have been said to have orgasmic experience at the same time.

Can a man and a woman have an orgasm at the same time?

It's possible but a lot of actors must be at play to achieve that.

The reason why it's hard though is the fact that woman tend to be shy to pleasure themselves for example to activate the clitoral spark plugs just before the black-red-yellow-black vaginal colour stage of orgasm. Men tend to hold everything to cook the woman and when they try to orgasm at the same time will have defrost and needing recooking.

If we are to ask what happens during sexual intercourse what will the vagina say?

What happens during sexual intercourse.

The vagina yarns to be opened enough to clinch - hold to something so that all the other processes can start as you can see from the list at the beginning everything depends on the vagina holding something inside without this all the essential processes cannot commence.

Holding a still dick code 72869838681.

Now if we are to have the requirement fulfilled then how long does it take to have all the correct processes in place

THE IMPORTANCE OF THE VAGINAL HOLD AND WHAT CAN BE DONE TO AFFECT THIS CONDITION.

If we are to ask what can be done to effect this condition there are three ways we can so this.

1] We must create a start.hold point inside the vagina. This point tells the vagina where to start. This point is a real reference to a point. We can ask a woman to put something larger like a cucumber inside her vagina and follow the simple steps below.

a] when object [cucumber] is inserted inside the vagina the woman must say;

create.start.hold

b] initiate.create.start.hold

c]repeat as needed intiate.create.start.hold

If we are to ask the vagina if it remembers the best hold it has surely that is something we can get an answer for.

Now say use best known configuration of hold to hold everything else

create.bestconfiguration.hold.start

Now you can ask the vagina to give this a name or number for example Davidbig or 2xxx choose any name you like.

Now you simply say install Davidbig or 2xxx and start from there

Now the vagina even though what is inside it is nothing or smaller it will use this known configuration to start the orgasm process.

Now say add everything else on top of that as if all is happening now.

addeverythingelseontopof.create.bestconfiguration.hold.start

Now the vagina must work from this best known configuration and work from there.

Now ask the vagina what was the best orgasm it had ever.

The vagina must easily tell you because this is as good as asking a person her favorite movie or color. The information is there and need not to be sought.

WHAT CAN BE DONE TO IMPROVE ON THE LAST KNOWN BEST ORGASMIC CLIMAX POINT?

Now ask what can be done to improve on the last known best orgasmic climax point?
The vagina will list everything in order:
1]increase attention given to a woman
2] increase hand [left] touch repeat if possible
3] increase kissing of the left check and not the right cheek
4] ask the correct questions
5] ask what if
6] ask what then
7] ask if then then what
8] ask what time
9] ask when time
10] ask if there is and stop
11] ask what if then stop
12] ask if you were mine then stop
13] ask if you were not mine then what
14] ask what then but why
15] ask why but why then
16] ask what if
17] ask when and as is
18] ask if not as is then what
19] ask what then it then
20] ask what if if not then
21] ever wonder kissing on the left cheek
22] ask what is and when is
23] if you were not mine then what
24] if you were mine but then stop
25] ask if what then what
26] ask what is when you can
27] ask what is when you can
28] ask if what then what again
29] if then what again
30] ask what is and what is not now that I know
31] if I didn't know then what and stop

32] if not then what is
33] if not then what is not
34] what is what and how is that so
35] if not then why is it like this
36] if not then why is it not like this
37] if you ask what if you can't ask
38] if you can then what
39] if you can't then what
40] if we can why wait
41] if we can't then what
42] when if not now
43] if not now then what
44] if not us then who
45] if not us why them
46] if us then why this and not that
47] if us then what
48] what is what of us
49] wat can we do
50] what is what and then stop
51] what is what of us and then stop
52] if we are to ask everything again then what
53] if we ask why then can we know why
54] if we ask can we expect a straight answer
55] if we are to join does that mean mutual agreement?
56] but if we are to ask can we get
57] if we ask why things happen they are do we expect the outcome
58] what is the role of your vagina in all this
59] can something else do all the work
60] can we start all over again if something does not work
61] Do you have the time
62] what can be expected of us if we start
63] can we stop once we have started
64] can we mingle later
65] what is that we must really do
66] can we ask if something goes wrong
67] can we choose when to start
68] if we can start who can stop us
69] if we can stop who can start us
70] why stop something like this

71] i think we cannot stop if we agree then let's continue until we both orgasm
72] in case you orgasm first then what can you sleep and I wake you up
73] if we orgasm together at the same time can that mean the end of sex
74] what if we both orgasm at the same time and we still want to go on who can start you or me
75] if we don't orgasm at the same time can this be the end of sex
76] If you orgasm first how can you make me orgasm as well without
77] if we start what can stop us
78] what is right to us
79] can we give up if this fails or find other means
80] can we start and try again later
81] if we stop what can be done to frustration
82] can we hand massage each other in case we can't do it by our brains
83] if we fail what would you prefer
84] if we fail what then
85] if we succeed then what
86] after orgasm what do you prefer a nap or a cuddle
87] sexually stimulate but had no orgasm then what? Can you start again after the great reset? and how?
88] I open my legs what's your response?
89]m i lick my lips [man] what is your response
90] i touch my groin [man] what is your response?
91] i finger your vagina what is your response?
92] I ogle your breasts what is your response?
93] I ogle your legs and groin what is your response
94] if I ask you to kiss me what is your response.

WHAT PARTS DOES A VAGINA HAVE AND THEIR ROLE IN ORGASM?

Now let's go deeper inside the vagina and ask what parts do you have and how they play a part in all this and in orgasm.
This is what the vagina would answer.
1] labia for external stimulation rubbing thighs and squeezing my thighs
2] clitoris for both internal and external stimuli. Clitoris is the ultimate orgasm driver. For every woman who cannot orgasm slap the clitoris to activate the clitoris' spark plugs.
3] the inner vagina that holds the shaft. This creates restore or memory points that can be used for the ultimate orgasmic experience. This is the beginning of orgasm because if this is lacking then whatever follows will not have the desired effect.
4] The outer vagina that includes the skin, pubic hairs, pussy lips and vulva opening. These are needed for external massage, touching, skin to skin contact etc
5] the rim of the vagina opening. The critical point in determine the hold.start point. Every woman's rings change as she grows older but rings can start big and become smaller and tight. A lot of things come into play.
6] the opening of the vagina. This is critical in that it determines the size of the hold. If mouth opening is small then the hold is greater but if mouth opening is wider the hold can be less.
But codes can be used to shrink or stretch the opening of the vagina.
Here is a list of vaginal opening codes and how to enforce them
7286983821
7286983328
7286983310
72869838480
72869831481
7296942384
7298488571
72685428581
7291238781
7287833441
7277841982
7286671148

7281802947
72774859001
72778924983
72786410182
727977485
7277864912
if we are to ask what to do with all these codes we can easily sat that we must tell woman's bodies to shrink to the best known configuration.
We can easily do this by telling the vagina to shrink to the right size
shrink.vagina.bestconfiguration.size.start
This command will tell your vagina to adopt the best known configuration so that it will have the best orgasm ever.
Now we can easily tell the female system that we want to use the best known opening size that can make it have the best orgasm.
Now that we have learnt how to configure the vagina system for best results let's get deeper into how the vagina actually performs an orgasm.

HOW THE VAGINA ACTUALLY PERFORMS AN ORGASM.

An orgasm is an end process resulting from attention and ending with a wonderful soul soothing and relaxing climax that resets everything to default predefined settings of a vagina.
Now let's look at how the inside pistols of the vagina are lubricated and works.
The vagina is the most none man-made complicated system on earth by far even the brain is easy to learn than the vagina.
This is because the brain tells you everything it does but the vagina cannot do the same.
Therefore, if we are to ask the vagina what that it does to get all wet and socked this is the answer.
I get attention above 90% for any lubrication to start.
A man must show me really love passion, attention, charm, charisma, passion for me to start the lubrication process.
Once that happens the chemical 1 s are released that sends messages to chemical 1 socket with commands to get wet and ready for the upcoming ulceration. When that happens, the sockets convert the received action potentials to nerve impulses that are then converted back to action potentials but ones that acts on the receptors rather than the inhibitors.
Knowing this is critical in that before or after arousal it is the same message that is sent to the vagina then to the brain of the woman but before arousal the message bounces off the inhibitors that don't have the right sockets therefore as good as not sent.
But during arousal the message are sent to the receptors once that have the converted sockets for receiving these. Once that happens that means that the required effect will be released. When this happens then the lubrication system is initiated. Once that has started now the frequency will be the determinate factor rather than the amount. That means that if a man gives the woman attention more frequently after the first then it's this frequency that determines the excretion of fluids in the vagina. The more the attention the more wet she becomes.
The process in play
The lubricant hormone LV is released from the vagina and sent to the chemical 1 receptor. These absorbs the lubricant hormone and pass them through the stripping of the binary numbers that are used as

identifying markers. When message is sent from one part of the body to the other the message is incapted using binary or non-binary numbers. Let's give a concrete example regarding lubrication.
Message from the vagina is sent to Chemical 1 receptors as makelubricant0 makelubricant1 makelubricant0 makelubricant1 when received in Chemical 1 receptors sockets the binary numbers are removed leaving the message makelubricant this is then rearranged before sending to become
1makelubricant 0makelubricant 1makelubricant 0makelubricant
This message is sent to Chemical 1 sockets and must fit this format for it to work.
Now let's see the whole process
When lubricant message is received in the sockets it makes it possible for the message to be decoded because the received message is the expected message as regarding the pre-defined apparatus system of the vagina.
The encoding simply adds binary at the beginning meaning the intended message is the second non-binary part.
When the message is sent at the beginning the message itself is not important but it's the binary that is important meaning nonfunctional message are to be decoded then encoded to get the meaning.
Now that the body receives the message the message is decoded and sent to the brain to be processed. Once received by the brain lubricant is released using the Chemical 1 socket to send corresponding action potentials to the part of the brain that release these lubricants. That means the chemical 1 socket release nerve hormones that carry messages to trigger the release of lubricants in the vagina. When this happens, we can now get lubricants.
But as said above from now on the amount depends on more attention rather than something else. The man must hit the right spots to increase the rhythm, frequencies that means asking the 40 critical questions cleverly in order and letting the next question cancel anything she says in response. This is the trick on other words you are actually programming her body to respond to you.
Now that we have looked at how lubrication works let's look at the most dreaded part of the vagina the clitoris.
The clitoris is a peanut size part of the vagina simply put that makes a woman climax without this no woman on earth would have been capable of orgasm.
The clitoris carries all the instructions and all the predefined system and

settings. That means all you need is inside the clitoris. Master the clitoris and make any woman on earth have an orgasm. But life is not as simple as this as you will see that a lot of forces come into play other than the clitoris that you might not know what is the problem if a woman fails to climax.
Now let's get deeper into the clitoris.
The clitoris is the most sensual part of the vagina in that it has so many nerve endings than the vagina itself.
The clitoris acts as the node of orgasm nerves. That means the central operating system or focal point of the vagina in terms of the orgasm. Once we know what the clitoris does then we can start to understand orgasm.
The clitoris has a hood that covers it. It is very sensitive to touch that long periods of touch can be painful rather than stimulus.
The clitoris has a billion nerve endings each coordinated for a specific purpose. Each nerve ending controls certain aspects of the vagina. In short, the clitoris is the central processing unit of the vagina and female reproduction organs and system of a woman.
The clitoris if known tells you what is wrong with the vagina. The clitoris asks questions.
1] what and why
2] where and how
3] why and where
4] when and what for
5] what for but why
6] what if
7] if what then what
8] if what then why
9] if then then what
10] what if i then what
11] if we then what
12] what is and why is it like that
13] if not then what
14] if what then why not
15] do you know this and stop
16] do you have this before and stop
17] what do you want then what
18] if you can then what
19] what can be done if not
20] if we can then what

21] if not then why
22] if why then why not
23] if not us then who
24] if not who then why not us
25] if we then what
26] what if then what
27] if we why not now
28] can we now and then what
29] if not us then who and why
30] who can if not us and why
31] if not us why others
32] why not us and who then
33] if not us why others
34] if not them why not us
35] if not us who and why
36] why them and not us
37] when and why
38] how and why
39] if not us then who and why
40] if we can't then who
41] if who then why not me [man] [woman]
42] if who then why not you [woman] [woman]
43] if we must then how
44] if we must then how
45] if not this way why not us
46] if not us then who
47] can we do it right now right here
48] if not why
49] why not now
50] why then and not now

Now that we have looked at all critical questions the clitoris must ask
we must go deeper and see the clitoris at work.
The clitoris commands the female reproductive organs from urinating
to arousal to climax.
The clitoris is responsible for a lot of functions in the body.
The clitoris tells a woman what to do
The clitoris commands a woman what to do
The clitoris gives a woman a reason to feel proud
The clitoris gives a woman pride
The clitoris gives a woman pleasure

The clitoris gives a woman every reason to live
The clitoris gives a woman a sense of self-worth.
The clitoris gives a woman a self worthy.
The clitoris tells a woman what to expect during clitoris stimulation
The clitoris tells a woman when to have an orgasm
The clitoris tells a woman how to have an orgasm.
The clitoris tells a woman how to achieve an orgasm.
The clitoris tells a woman when to have an orgasm.
The clitoris tells a woman about the state of things and how to improve them.
The clitoris tells a woman how to respond to attention by men or other women.
If we are to ask what can happen during clitoral stimulation the brain will tell you that the clitoris will get really excited and change.
Once enlarged then we can expect it to have a lot of traffic inside it as things get heated up.
Now we can separate each activity as it happens.
Let's look how stimulation of the clitoris work.
The clitoris gets aroused by chemicals mainly Chemical 1 the first class or category these acts directly on the clitoris sockets responsible for stimuli.
Once that happens the clitoris receives messages with binary first meaning nonfunctional messages. The sockets remove the binary to get to the bottom of things meaning getting to the meaning of the things.
Once that is done the message is revealed and sent to the brain to be processed but first since message is important the message is still assigned binary numbers but the binary is secondary.
The message is then sent to the brain.
Once in the brain the message is processed and the nerve impulses and their corresponding action potentials are activated.
Once that is done the message is decoded and the commands are sent to the receptor's sockets fitted in and the agents sent to the correct functions.
That means the clitoris is further aroused just by receiving and sending messages. This is because electromagnetic wave stimulation is involved as is in electromagnetic internisonents where electromagnetic wave causes vaginal ulceration to trigger rhythm stimulation.
Once this has happened then we can expect the clitoris to start its own ulceration 7286984832 and to swell as blood flows in delivering and extracting messages.

This together with vaginal stimulation trigger initiation of orgasm in woman. Again, as a reminder unless there is need for extra electromagnetic internisonent then slapping of the clit is a must to activate the clitoral spark plug.
Once this is done then it's only a matter of time before orgasm sets in.

PROCESSES INSIDE THE VAGINA CALLED SQUANKS.

Now let's look at the inside of the vagina process that are called the squanks.
The Squanks.
As the name suggest these depends on the hold by the vagina from the rim to the inside trunk. The greatest the hold the better the squanks.
If we are to ask the vagina what happens inside it this is the answer we get.
Inside the vagina once the hold is established then everything else follows easily. According to the vagina after the grip and hold is established then everything else follows a pre-defined sequence.
1] Squanks are activated.
2] squinks are activated
3] squinkos are activated
4] squinkozs are activated
5] squinkitz are activated
6] squinkitzs are activated
7] squinkitzo are activated
8] squinkitzos are activated
9] squinkitzot are activated
10] squinkitzots are activated
11] squinkotzots are activated
12] squinkotzotsz are activated
13] squinkotzotszo are activated
14] squinkotzotszot are activated
15] squinkotzotszotnz are activated
16] squinkotzotszotnzw are activated
17] squinkotzotszotnzwo are activated
18] squinkotzotszotnzwots are activated
19] squinkotzotwsrstz are activated
20] squinkotzotwsrstzo are activated
21] squinkotzotwsrstzow are activated
Now that all the squantz are activated we can do this by way of codes for each
1] 72869848321
2] 72869848385
3] 72869848381

4] 728698483814
5] 7286983851684
6] 72869838551783
7] 72869838778641
8] 72879848321084
9] 72984838649821
10] 72987884324868
11] 7298718364853
12]7248687118528
13]727978028418
14] 727868524800
15] 72797283289
16] 72785868283
17]721849828671
18] 72728685841
19] 7271738690
20] 7248566384
21] 72798648381
Now after everything is achieved we can expect the next set of activities to happen.
The vagina will go through all the 21-process stage by stages depending on frequency.

SPECIFIC QUESTIONS POSED TO THE VAGINA REGARDING ORGASM.

Now all we need to do is to ask the vagina specific questions related to orgasm.

1] If the shaft is right what combinations can give you the most enormous orgasm ever? The answer is all in that sequence from 1 to 21 without skipping a stage.

2] if we are to ask what can severely go wrong the answer is; if the hold is missing everything can go wrong.

3] Now if we are to ask what give the fastest orgasm ever the vagina will answer combinations

1,3,7,9 and 21 in that order

4] if we are to ask the vagina what makes you squit something others can't do what is the response to this?

The answer clipping of the shaft meaning end of vagina compressing the shaft [dick] and opening squeezing as well when this happens that means the vagina acts as a compressor to the bladder that contains fluids in a woman meaning squirting of the urinary valve as liquids are squeezed by the compressed vagina but squirting in this way might not be stimulating itself. The stimulation can come from the compressed vaginal rhythms.

5] What makes a woman want sex and then orgasm?

The answer constant attention makes woman want to be fucked because this trigger the need to orgasm.

6] If a woman constantly wants sex what does that mean?

Constantly craving for sex can be a result of increased attention. Blondes get aroused fast and quickly and you are likely to score from a blond than a brunette. But depends on other factors as well.

7] If we are to ask the vagina why sometimes it does not orgasm what is the answer?

The answer is that tiredness in women can make the body save energy especially if she gets up early. Women with hard schedules and tight deadlines are ones who often fail to have an orgasm more often than less hard-working women. Some women can fail to orgasm if they hold grudges with their counterparts or if they harbor a secret or think that their partner harbor a secret.

8] What makes women horny alone if we ask the vagina what is the answer?

Women often feel horny if hormones are increased and what increase hormones can be anything.

9] What can be said about hormones sex, orgasm and lust? Is there a link to all this?

It depends on woman as some have good hormones that make the whole process last long or fast depending on circumstances.

10] If we are to ask why women can't orgasm after menstruation the answer is that the vaginal biological clock will have died. All the process above will have become worn out so that hold is missing therefore everything else dies or malfunctions.

GIVING WOMEN A SECOND CHANCE BY CREATING A BEST KNOW GOOD GONFIGURATION

But creating a best good known configuration orgasm point can give women the chance to orgasm again because this is the only thing that malfunctions to render a vagina after menstruation useless.
The commands needed.
create.bestknownconfiguration.hold.start
initiate.create.bestknownconfiguration.hold.start
activate.initiate.create.bestknownconfiguration.hold.start
Once all this is set up a woman can use this to masturbate if sex has become painful in old age.

A QUICK LOOK AT MALE EJACUALTION

Now let's look at what happens to the male ejaculation.
A man can easily ejaculate if he has sperms inside his sacks. This is the only thing that is needed: sperm.
If there is no sperm then ejaculation can still happen but without the added excitement.
First like females' males can; -
create.bestknownconfiguration.ejacualtion.start
To kickstart the ejaculation process but overall the process for a man is simple as compared to that of a female.
Males need only to manufacture enough sperms enough to want to fuck anything that moves even cracks in the rocks.
This is the process.
When sperm fills 90% of sack volume a nerve impulse message is sent to the brain. This is attached to binary numbers as a nonfunctional command.
When received in the brain by the nerve impulse receptors the message is stripped off the binary numbers and encoding with binary as a secondary function.
That means the message now has priority. The message is sent to the brain action potential receptors only after being converted into action potentials from nerve impulses.
Now the message is decoded and the right brain stimuli to effect a sexual response is effected. The man now easily will get arousal from seeing a woman or even her legs can trigger the need to fuck.
But constant frustration or rejection can have the opposite effect in that man can ignore potential mates just by past rejections.
A man unlike a female need not attention but can easily use his hand and memory on sight stimuli to effect ejaculation easily than what a woman would.
The ejaculation process in detail.

ORGASM AND EJACULATION AS THE ANSWER TO CREATION AND GOD'S PLAN.

Once penetration is achieved it becomes a push and pull system. The man pushes thrusting hard to effect hold and grip as a woman's vagina tightens hard. The thrusting is the most effective way of achieving ejaculation. The faster and the tight the hold the fast the ejaculation. Thrusting sends messages to the balls sockets to compress and ejaculate all fluids in response to the thrusting.

If thrusting is achieved the pressure keep piling in the ball's sacks to such an extent that everything will be squeezed out.

That means after when the sacks are drained air replaces the fluid and resets the system as it escapes the sacks valve that introduced the sperm in the ducts in the first place.

This activates the reset switch that sets everything to original point before ejaculation and before building up of sperm.

Now let's look at malfunction to the man's system.

Impotent, old age and a lot of other functions like being cheated upon or artificial blocking can render a man as impotent to ejaculation. But unless it's a serious injury everything is temporary and can reset itself or after talking about the issue.

Now you can see that the mating orgasm and ejaculation between lovers etc is a very complicated process but the answer to creation and God's plan.

Attention is all that is needed to ensure the survival of mankind. Man must pay attention to the woman to get laid and for her to orgasm and for him to ejaculate.

All it takes is a hie I am interested in you and I promise I will give you so much attention you will literally come in my face.

The end.

40 Steps to make any woman have the best orgasm.

The Ultimate recipe to get a woman orgasm.
1] Maintain and look at her in the eyes. The opening.
2] The invite
3] The internal search.
4] ...

WOMEN GET A DESIGNER VAGINA USING THESE CODES.

See other previous books in the series.

MEN GET A DESIGNER PENIS USING THESE CODES.

See other previous books in the series.

ABOUT DAVID GOMADZA

Visit www.twofuture.world